The Ultimate Bread Machine Cookbook Guide

50 easy and affordable recipes for your healthy bread machine

Sofia Bishop

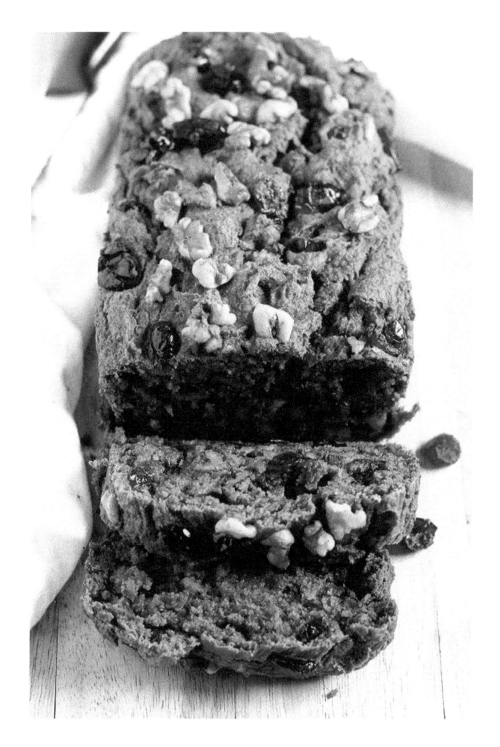

COPYRIGHT

Table of Contents

Peanut Butter and Jelly Bread

Preparation Time: 10 minutes

1½-Pound Loaf

Ingredients:

· 1½ tablespoons vegetable oil

· 1 cup of water

· ½ cup blackberry jelly

· ½ cup peanut butter

· 1 teaspoon salt

· 1 tablespoon white sugar

· 2 cups of bread flour

· 1 cup whole-wheat flour

· 1½ teaspoons active dry yeast

Directions:

1.Put everything in your bread machine pan.

2.Select the basic setting.

3.Press the start button.

4.Take out the pan when done and set aside for 5minutes.

Nutrition:

· Calories: 193

· Carbohydrates: 11 g

· Fat: 9 g

· Cholesterol: 0 mg

· Protein: 4 g

· Fiber: 2 g

· Sugars: 11 g

· Sodium: 244 mg

· Potassium: 1 mg

Low-Carb Bagel

Preparation Time: 1 hour

1½-Pound Loaf

Ingredients:

· 1 cup protein powder, unflavored

· 1/3 cup coconut flour

· 1 teaspoon baking powder

· ½ teaspoon sea salt

· ¼ cup ground flaxseed

· 1/3 cup sour cream

· 1½ eggs

Seasoning topping :

· 1 teaspoon dried parsley

· 1 teaspoon dried oregano

· 1 teaspoon dried minced onion

· ½ teaspoon garlic powder

· ½ teaspoon dried basil

· ½ teaspoon sea salt

Directions:

1.Preheat the oven to 350° F.

2.In a mixer, blend sour cream and eggs until well combined.

3.Whisk together the flaxseed, salt, baking powder, Protein: powder, and coconut flour in a bowl.

4.Mix the dry ingredients until it becomes wet ingredients. Make sure it is well blended.

5.Whisk the topping seasoning together in a small bowl. Set aside.

6.Grease 2 donut pans that can contain six donuts each.

7.Sprinkle pan with about 1 teaspoon. Topping seasoning and evenly pour batter into each.

8.Sprinkle the top of each bagel evenly with the rest of the seasoning mixture.

9.Bake in the oven for 25 minutes, or until golden brown.

Nutrition:

· Calories: 174

· Sodium: 267 mg

· Fat: 6.1 g

· Carbohydrates: 4.2 g

· Protein: 1½ g

Puri Bread

Preparation Time: 1 hour

1-Pound Loaf

Ingredients:

· 1 cup almond flour, sifted

· ½ cup of warm water

· 2 tablespoons clarified butter

· 1 cup olive oil for frying

· Salt to taste

Directions:

1.Salt the water and add the flour.

2.Make some holes in the center of the dough and pour warm clarified butter.

3.Knead the dough and let stand for 15 minutes, covered.

4.Shape into six balls.

5.Flatten the balls into six thin rounds using a rolling pin.

6.Heat enough oil to cover a round frying pan completely.

7.Place a puri in it when hot.

8.Fry for 1 second on each side.

9.Place on a paper towel.

10. Repeat with the rest of the puri and serve.

Nutrition:

· Calories: 176

· Fat: 3 g

· Carbohydrates: 6 g

· Protein: 3 g

· Sodium: 80 mg

Bread Roll

Preparation Time: 1 hour

1-Pound Loaf

Ingredients:

· 2 tablespoons coconut oil, melted

· 6 tablespoons coconut flour

· ¼ teaspoon baking soda

· 1 tablespoon Italian seasoning

· ½ teaspoon salt

· 2 tablespoons gelatin

· 6 tablespoons hot water

Directions:

1.Preheat the oven to 300° F (150°C).

2.Mix the coconut oil, coconut flour, and baking soda.

3.In a separate bowl, whisk together the gelatin and hot water to create your gelatin egg.

4.Pour the gelatin egg into the coconut flour mixture and combine well.

5.Add in the Italian seasoning and salt to taste (you can taste the mixture to see if you want to add more) and mix well into a dough.

6.Use your hands to form 2 small rolls from the dough, place the rolls on a baking tray lined with parchment paper, and bake in the oven for 40-50 minutes until the outside of each roll is lightly browned and crispy like you'd typically find in a regular breadroll.

7.Let the rolls cool down before serving so that the gelatin sets a bit and can hold the roll together. Enjoy at room temperature with some ghee or coconutoil.

8.This recipe can be doubled, tripled, etc. If you want to make more AIP bread rolls at the sametime.

Nutrition:

· Calories: 290

· Sodium: 320 mg

· Fat: 23.6 g

· Carbohydrates: 11 g

· Protein: 33.5 g

Bacon Breakfast Bagels

Preparation Time: 2 hours

2-PoundLoaf

Ingredients:

· Bagels

· ¾ cup (61 g) almond flour

· 1 teaspoon Xanthan gum

· 1 large egg

· 1½ cups grated mozzarella

· 2 tablespoons cream cheese

· toppings

· 1 tablespoon butter, melted

· 1 teaspoon salt

· Sesame seeds to taste

· fillings

· 2 tablespoons pesto

· 2 tablespoons cream cheese

· 1 cup arugula leaves

· 6 slices grilled streaky bacon

Directions:

1. Preheat oven to 390° F.

2.In a bowl mix together the almond flour and Xanthan gum. Then add the egg and mix together until well combined. Set a side. It will look like a doughy ball.

3.In a pot over a medium-low heat slowly melt the creamcheese and mozzarella together and remove from heat once melted. This can be done in the microwave as well.

4.Add your melted cheese mix to the almond flour mix and knead until well combined. The Mozzarella mix will stick together in a bit of a ball but don't worry, persist with it. It will all combine well eventually. It's important to get the Xanthan gum incorporated through the cheese mix. Suppose the dough gets too tough to work, place in microwave for few seconds to warm and repeat until you have some thing that resembles a dough.

5.Split your dough into 3 pieces and roll into round logs. If you have a donut pan, place yourlogs into the pan. If not, make circles with each logand join together and place on a baking tray. Try to make sure you have nice little circles. The other way to do this is to make a ball and flattens lightly on the baking tray and cut a circle out of the middle if you have a small cookie cutter.

6.Melt your butter and brush over the top of your bagels and sprinkle sesame seeds or your topping of choice. The butter should help the seeds stick. Garlic and onion powder or cheesemake nice additions if you have them for savory bagels.

7.Place bagels in the oven for about 11½ minutes. Keep an eye on them. The topsshouldgo golden brown.

8.Take the bagels out of the oven and allow to cool.

9.If you like your bagels toasted, cut them in half lengthwise and place back in the oven until slightly golden and toasty.

10. Spread bagel with cream chease, cover in pesto, add a few arugula leaves and top with your crispybacon (or your filling of choice.)

Nutrition:

· Calories: 605

· Fat: 50 g

· Carbohydrates: 57 g

· Protein: 30.1 g

· Sodium: 295 mg

Hot Dog Buns

Preparation Time: 1 hour

1-Pound Loaf

Ingredients:

· 1¼ cups almond flour

· 5 tablespoons psyllium husk powder

· 1 teaspoon sea salt

· 2 teaspoons baking powder

· 1¼ cups boiling water

· 2 teaspoons lemon juice

· 3 eggs whites

Directions:

1.Preheat the oven to 350° F

2.In a bowl, put all dry ingredients and mix well.

3.Add boiling water, lemon juice, and egg whites into the dry mixture and whisk until combined.

4.Mould the dough into ten portions and roll into buns.

5.Transfer into the preheated oven and cook for 40 to 50 minutes on the lower oven rack.

6.Check for doneness and remove it.

7.Top with desired toppings and hot dogs.

8. Serve.

Nutrition:

· Calories: 214

· Fat: 1½ g

· Carbohydrates: 4 g

· Protein: 4 g

· Sodium: 242 mg

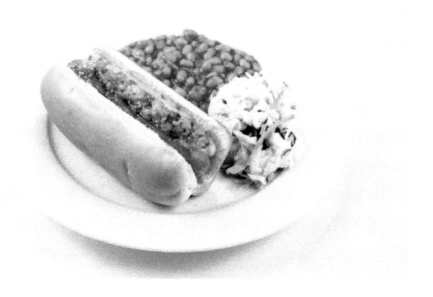

Paleo Coconut Bread

Preparation Time: 1 hour

1½ -Pound Loaf

Ingredients:

· ½ cup coconut flour

· ¼ cup almond milk (unsweetened)

· ¼ cup coconut oil (melted)

· 6 eggs

· ¼ teaspoon baking soda

· ¼ teaspoon salt

Directions:

1.Preheat the oven to 350° F.

2.Prepare a (1½ x 4) bread pan with parchment paper.

3.In a bowl, combine salt, baking soda, and coconut flour.

4.Combine the oil, milk, and eggs in another bowl.

5.Gradually add the wet ingredients into the dry ingredients and mix well.

6.Pour the mixture into the prepared pan.

7.Bake for 40 to 50 minutes.

8.Cool, slice, and serve.

Nutrition:

· Calories: 191

· Fat: 11 g

· Carbohydrates: 3.4 g

· Protein: 4.2 g

· Sodium: 220 mg

Healthy Low Carb Bread

Preparation Time: 1 hour

1½-Pound Loaf

Ingredients:

· 2/3 cup coconut flour

· 2/3 cup coconut oil (softened not melted)

· 9 eggs

· 2 teaspoons cream of tartar

· ¾ teaspoon Xanthan gum

· 1 teaspoon baking soda

· ¼ teaspoon salt

Directions:

1.Preheat the oven to 350° F.

2.Grease a pound pan with 1 to 2 teaspoons. Melted coconut oil and place it in the freezer to harden.

3.Add eggs into a bowl and mix for 2 minutes with a hand mixer.

4.Add coconut oil into the eggs and mix.

5.Add dry ingredients to a second bowl and whisk until mixed.

6.Put the dry ingredients into the egg mixture and mix on low speed with a hand mixer until dough is formed and the mixture is incorporated.

7. Add the dough into the prepared pound pan, transfer it into the preheated oven, and bake for 35 minutes.

8.Take out the bread pan from the oven.

9.Cool, slice, and serve.

Nutrition:

· Calories: 229

· Carbohydrates: 6 g

· Sodium: 60 mg

· Fat: 25.5 g

· Protein: 4 g

Spicy Bread

Preparation Time: 1 hour

1½-Pound Loaf

Ingredients:

· ½ cup coconut flour

· 6 eggs

· 3 large jalapenos, sliced

· 4 ounces' turkey bacon, sliced

· ½ cup ghee

· ¼ teaspoon baking soda

· ¼ teaspoon salt

· ¼ cup of water

Directions:

1.Preheat the oven to 400°F.

2.Cut bacon and jalapenos on a baking tray and roast for 1 1/4 minutes.

3.Flip and bake for five more minutes.

4.Remove seeds from the jalapenos.

5.Place jalapenos and bacon pounds in a food processor and blend until smooth.

6.In a bowl, add ghee, eggs, and ¼-cup water. Mix well.

7. Then add some coconut flour, baking soda, and salt. Stir to mix.

8.Add bacon and jalapeno mix.

9.Grease the pound pan with ghee.

10. Pour batter into the pound pan.

11. Bake for 40 minutes.

Enjoy.

Nutrition:

· Calories: 240

· Sodium: 180 mg

· Carbohydrates: 7 g

· Fat: 1g

Fluffy Paleo Bread

Preparation Time: 1 hour

2-Pound Loaf

Ingredients:

· 1¼ cups almond flour

· 5 eggs

· 1 teaspoon lemon juice

· 1/3 cup avocado oil

· 1 dash black pepper

· ½ teaspoon sea salt

· 3 to 4 tablespoons tapioca flour

· 1 to 2 teaspoons poppy seed

· ¼ cup ground flaxseed

· ½ teaspoon baking soda

· top with:

· poppy seeds

· pumpkin seeds

Directions:

1.Preheat the oven to 350° F.

2.Line a baking pan with parchment paper and set aside.

3. In a bowl, add eggs, avocado oil, and lemon juice and whisk until combined.

4.In another bowl, add tapioca flour, almond flour, baking soda, flaxseed, black pepper, and poppy seed. Mix.

5.Add the lemon juice mixture into the flour mixture and mix well.

6.Add the batter into the prepared pound pan and top with extra pumpkin seeds and poppy seeds.

7.Cover pound pan and transfer into the prepared oven, and bake for 1 minute. Remove cover and bake until an inserted knife comes out clean after about 15 minutes.

8.Remove from oven and cool.

9.Slice and serve.

Nutrition:

· Calories: 190

· Sodium: 190 mg

· Fat: 2 g

· Carbohydrates: 4.4 g

German Pumpernickel Bread

Preparation Time: 10 minutes

2-Pound Loaf

Ingredients:

· 1½ tablespoons vegetable oil

· 1½ cups warm water

· 3 tablespoons cocoa

· 1/3 cup molasses

· 1½ teaspoons salt

· 1 tablespoon caraway seeds

· 1 cup rye flour

· 1½ cups of bread flour

· 1½ tablespoons wheat gluten

· 1 cup whole wheat flour

· 2½ teaspoons bread machine yeast

Directions:

1.Put everything in your bread machine.

2.Select the primary cycle.

3.Hit the start button.

4.Transfer bread to a rack for cooling once done.

Nutrition:

· Calories: 189

· Carbohydrates: 22.4 g

· Total Fat 2.3 g

· Cholesterol: 0mg

· Protein: 3 g

· Sodium: 360 mg

European Black Bread

Preparation Time: 10 minutes

1½-Pound Loaf

Ingredients:

· 1 cup of water

· ¾ teaspoon cider vinegar

· ½ cup rye flour

· 1½ cups flour

· 1 tablespoon margarine

· ¼ cup of oat bran

· 1 teaspoon salt

· 1½ tablespoons sugar

· 1 teaspoon dried onion flakes

· 1 teaspoon caraway seed

· 1 teaspoon yeast

· 2 tablespoons unsweetened cocoa

Directions:

1.Put everything in your bread machine.

2.Now select the basic setting.

3.Hit the start button.

4.Transfer bread to a rack for cooling once done.

Nutrition:

· Calories: 191

· Carbohydrates: 22 g

· Total fat: 1.7 g

· Cholesterol: 0mg

· Protein: 3 g

· Sugar: 2 g

· Sodium: 247 mg

French Baguettes

Preparation Time: 25 minutes

1½-Pound Loaf

Ingredients:

· 1¼ cups warm water

· 3½ cups bread flour

· 1 teaspoon salt

· 1 package active dry yeast

Directions:

1.Place ingredients in the bread machine. Select the dough cycle. Hit the start button.

2.When the dough cycle is finished, remove it with floured hands and cut in half on a well-floured.

3.Take each half of the dough and roll it to make a pound about 1½ inches long in the shape of French bread.

4.Place on a greased baking sheet and cover with a towel.

5.Let rise until doubled, about 1 hour.

6.Preheat oven to 450° F (210° C).

7.Bake until golden brown, turning the pan around once halfway during baking.

8.Transfer the loaves to a rack.

Nutrition:

· Calories: 161

· Carbohydrates: 42 g

· Total Fat 0.6 g

· Cholesterol: 0 mg

· Protein: 6 g

· Fiber: 1.7 g

· Sugars: 0.1 g

· Sodium: 240 mg

Portuguese Sweet Bread

Preparation Time: 10 minutes

1-Pound Loaf

Ingredients:

· 1 egg beaten

· 1 cup milk

· 1/3 cup sugar

· 2 tablespoons margarine

· 3 cups bread flour

· ¾ teaspoon salt

· 2½ teaspoons active dry yeast

Directions:

1.Place everything into your bread machine.

2.Select the sweet bread setting. Hit the start button.

3.Transfer the loaves to a rack for cooling once done.

Nutrition:

· Calories: 179

· Carbohydrates: 24 g

· Total Fat: 11½ g

· Cholesterol: 1 mg

· Protein: 3 g

· Fiber: 0g

· Sugars: 4 g

· Sodium: 180 mg

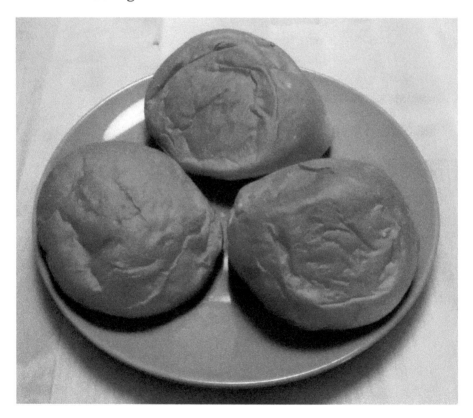

Italian Bread

Preparation Time: 2 hours

1-Pound Loaf

Ingredients:

· 1 tablespoon of light brown sugar

· 4 cups all-purpose flour, unbleached

· 1½ teaspoons of salt

· 11/3 cups + 1 tablespoon warm water

· 1 package active dry yeast

· 1½ teaspoons of olive oil

· 1 egg

· 2 tablespoons cornmeal

Directions:

1.Place flour, brown sugar, 1/3 cup warm water, salt, olive oil, and yeast in your bread machine. Select the dough cycle. Hit the start button.

2.Deflate your dough. Turn it on a floured surface.

3.Form two loaves from the dough.

4.Keep them on your cutting board. The seam side should be down. Sprinkle some cornmeal on your board.

5.Place a damp cloth on your loaves to cover them.

6.Wait for 40 minutes. The volume should double.

7. In the meantime, preheat your oven to 190° C.

8.Beat 1 tablespoon of water and an egg in a bowl.

9.Brush this mixture on your loaves.

10. Make an extended cut at the center of your loaves with a knife.

11. Shake your cutting board gently, making sure that the loaves do not stick.

12. Now slide your loaves on a baking sheet.

13. Bake in your oven for about 35 minutes.

Nutrition:

· Calories: 165

· Carbohydrates: 1.6 g

· Total Fat: 0.9 g

· Cholesterol: 9 mg

· Protein: 3.1 g

· Fiber: 1 g

· Sugars: 1g

Pita Bread

Preparation Time: 1 hour

1½-PoundLoaf

Ingredients:

· 3 cups of all-purpose flour

· 1½ cups warm water

· 1 tablespoon of vegetable oil

· 1 teaspoon salt

· 1½ teaspoons active dry yeast

· 1 active teaspoon white sugar

Directions:

1.Place all the ingredients in your bread pan.

2.Select the dough setting. Hit the start button.

3.The machine beeps after the dough rises adequately.

4.Turn the dough on a floured surface.

5.Roll and stretch the dough gently into a 1½ inch rope.

6.Cut into eight pieces with a knife.

7.Now roll each piece into a ball. It should be smooth.

8.Roll each ball into a 7-inch circle. Keep covered with a towel on a floured top for 30 minutes for the pita to rise. It should get puffy slightly.

9. Preheat your oven to 260° C.

10. Keep the pitas on your wire cake rack. Transfer to the oven rack directly.

11. Bake the pitas for 5 minutes. They should be puffed. The top should start to brown.

12. Take out from the oven. Keep the pitas immediately in a sealed paper bag. You can also cover using a damp kitchen towel.

13. Split the top edge or cut it into half once the pitas are soft. You can also have the whole pitas if you want.

Nutrition:

· Calories: 191

· Carbohydrates: 37 g

· Total Fat: 3g

· Cholesterol: 0mg

· Protein: 5g

· Fiber: 1g

· Sugars: 1g

· Sodium: 243mg

· Potassium: 66mg

Syrian Bread

Preparation Time: 1 hour

1½-Pound Loaf

Ingredients:

· 2 tablespoons vegetable oil

· 1 cup of water

· 1½ teaspoon salt

· ½ teaspoon white sugar

· 1½ teaspoons active dry yeast

· 3 cups all-purpose flour

Directions:

1. Put everything in your bread machine pan.

2. Select the dough cycle. Hit the start button.

3. Preheat your oven to 475 degrees F.

4. Turn to dough on a lightly floured surface once done.

5. Divide it into eight equal pieces. Form them into rounds.

6. Take a damp cloth and cover the rounds with it.

7.Now roll the dough into flat thin circles. They should have a diameter of around 1½ inches.

8.Cook in your preheated baking sheets until they are golden brown and puffed.

Nutrition:

· Calories: 169

· Carbohydrates: 36 g

· Total Fat 5 g

· Protein: 5 g

· Fiber: 1 g

· Sugar: 0 g

· Sodium: 360 mg

· Potassium: 66 mg

Ethiopian Milk and Honey Bread

Preparation Time: 10 minutes

1-Pound Loaf

Ingredients:

· 3 tablespoons honey

· 1 cup + 1 tablespoon milk

· 3 cups bread flour

· 3 tablespoons melted butter

· 2 teaspoons active dry yeast

· 1½ teaspoon salt

Directions:

1.Add everything to the pan of your bread

2.Select the white bread or basic setting and the medium crust setting.

3.Hit the start button.

4.Take out your hot pound once it is done.

5.Keep on your wire rack for cooling.

6.Slice your bread once it is cold and serve.

Nutrition:

· Calories: 189

· Carbohydrates: 1 g

· Total Fat 3.1 g

· Cholesterol: 0 mg

· Protein: 2.4 g

· Fiber: 0.6 g

· Sugars: 3.3 g

· Sodium: 362 mg

Swedish Cardamom Bread

Preparation Time: 1 hour

1-Pound Loaf

Ingredients:

· ¼ cup of sugar

· ¾ cup of warm milk

· ¾ teaspoon cardamom

· ½ teaspoon salt

· ¼ cup of softened butter

· 1 egg

· 2¼ teaspoons bread machine yeast

· 3 cups all-purpose flour

· 5 tablespoons milk for brushing

· 2 tablespoons sugar for sprinkling

Directions:

1.Put everything (except milk for brushing and sugar for sprinkling) in the pan of your bread machine.

2.Select the dough cycle. Hit the start button. You should have an elastic and smooth dough once the process is complete. It should be double in size.

3.Transfer to a lightly floured surface.

4.Now divide into three balls. Set aside for 5minutes.

5.Roll all the balls into long ropes of around 1 inch.

6.Braid the shapes. Pinch ends under securely and keeps on a cookie sheet. You can also divide your dough into two balls. Smooth them and keep them on your bread pan.

7.Brush milk over the braid. Sprinkle sugar lightly.

8.Now bake in your oven for 25 minutes at 375° F (190° C).

9. Take a foil and cover for the final 5minutes. It's prevents over-browning.

10. Transfer to your cooling rack.

Nutrition:

· Calories: 185

· Carbohydrates: 22 g

· Total Fat: 7g

· Cholesterol: 1mg

· Protein: 3g

· Fiber: 1 g

· Sugars: 3g

Fiji Sweet Potato Bread

Preparation Time: 10 minutes

1-Pound Loaf

Ingredients:

· 1 teaspoon vanilla extract

· ½ cup of warm water

· 4 cups flour

· 1 cup sweet mashed potatoes

· 2 tablespoons softened butter

· ½ teaspoon cinnamon

· 1½ teaspoons salt

· 1/3 cup brown sugar

· 2 tablespoons powdered milk

· 2 teaspoons yeast

Directions:

1.Add everything in the pan of your bread.

2.Select the white bread and the crust you want.

3.Hit the start button.

4.Set aside on wire racks for cooling before slicing.

Nutrition:

· Calories: 182

· Carbohydrates: 21 g

· Fat: 5 g

· Protein: 4 g

· Fiber: 1 g

· Sugar 3 g

· Sodium: 360 mg

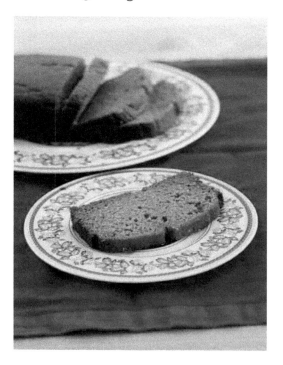

Sourdough Baguette

Preparation Time: 1 hour

2 -Pound Loaf

Ingredients:

· 3¼ cups bread flour

· 1 cup sourdough starter

· 1 cup water

· 1¾ teaspoons fine sea salt

Directions:

1.Mix the starter, flour, water, and salt. Mix with a spatula until you get a shaggy dough. Cover using a kitchen towel and leave for 30 minutes.

2.Knead for 5minutes until the dough starts to feel smooth. Scrape the sides of the bowl and lightly oil the insides. Form a ball and put it in the bowl. Cover again and leave for 2-4 hours to double in size.

3.Punch the dough down on a floured surface. Make a rectangle from the dough and fold it in thirds to the middle beginning from one short side. Pinch the ends closed. Put the dough back into the bowl, cover, and leave for 30 minutes. Repeat this step again.

4.Divide your dough evenly into 3 pieces.

5.Put them on a floured work surface to form baguettes. Line a rimless baking sheet with a piece of parchment paper and transfer the baguettes onto it. Cover with a kitchen towel and leave for 30 minutes.

6. Meanwhile, preheat the oven to 450°F. Put a baking sheet on the middle rack and a cast-iron skillet on the rack below. Prepare a cup of ice cubes.

7.When baguettes have almost doubled in size, cut few slashes on their tops with a knife. Lightly dampen them and place them on the hot baking sheet. Pour the ice cubes into the skillet and close the oven door. Set to 400° F and bake for 1 minute. Bake for longer if you want your crust deep colored.

8.Take them out and let them cool for 30 minutes before slicing.

Nutrition:

· Calories: 175

· Carbohydrates: 24 g

· Fat: 0 g

· Protein:2 g

· Sodium: 360 g

Classic French Baguette

Preparation Time: 30 min. + 11 hours

2-Pound Loaf

Ingredients:

For the poolish:

· ¾ cup bread flour

· 6 tablespoons + 1 teaspoon filtered water, warm 90°F

· ¼ teaspoon active dry yeast

· For the final dough:

· 1¾ cups bread flour

· ½ cup all-purpose flour

· ½ cup + 3 tablespoons filtered water, warm 90°F

· ¼ teaspoon active dry yeast

· 1¼ teaspoon kosher salt

Directions:

1.Make a poolish in advance. Mix all of the ingredients in a large bowl. Cover it with plastic wrap and leave for 1½ – 5hours.

2.Then, add all of the ingredients for the dough to the poolish. Stir well to combine. Knead it with your hands until you get a shaggy dough and leave for 30 minutes covered with plastic wrap.

3.Next, dampen your hands and pull on and stretch up one side of the dough, then fold down over the top of the dough. Repeat for each side after the rotating bowl 90 degrees when the last side is done. Cover and leave for 30 minutes. Repeat this process four times.

4.Meanwhile, prepare the equipment: set one oven rack in the middle and another at the bottom position. Put an upside-down sheet pan on the middle rack. Preheat the oven to 500° F for 1 hour. Flour a lint-free towel and line an undimmed baking sheet with parchment paper.

5.Divide the dough into two equal portions by cutting it. Place them on a lightly floured surface. Form a rectangle from one piece of dough and carefully stretch out the short ends. Fold every short end to the center, press it down with your fingertips to seal. Do the same with every long end to create a seam in the dough. Repeat this process with another piece. Cover both pieces with plastic wrap and leave for 5minutes.

6.Place one-piece seam side up and press it into a thin rectangle. Start folding down your dough (½") and sealing it with fingerprints, beginning from the top-left edge. Work across the top in the same way. Create a tight log by continuing folding down on the dough and sealing it. You should get a thin, tight log. Flip it seam side down. Roll your dough evenly into a long thin snake shape using both hands. Work it into a 1" baguette. Transfer it onto the prepared floured towel. Create the folds for holding the dough's shape by pushing a towel up on both sides of the baguette. Repeat all the steps for the second portion. Cover the baguettes with plastic wrap and leave for 1 hour to rise.

7.Carefully flip the baguettes onto parchment paper, seam side down. Cut 4-5 ¼" deep diagonal slashes on the top of the baguettes with a sharp knife.

8.Prepare a small bowl filled with 2 cups of ice cubes. Open the oven and gently slide the whole piece of parchment paper with the baguettes onto the preheated sheet pan. Pour ice into the preheated skillet and close the oven door immediately. Turn the temperature down to 475° F and bake for about 25-40 minutes depending on what crust you want for your baguettes.

9. Take them out of the oven and transfer them to a cooling rack. Let them cool for 30 minutes before slicing.

Nutrition:

· Calories: 172

· Carbohydrates:15 g

· Fat: 0 g

· Protein: 3 g

· Sodium: 360 mg

Alternative French Baguettes

Preparation Time: 10 minutes +2 h.

1½ -Pound Loaf

Ingredients:

· olive oil, for greasing

· 3¾ cups strong white bread flour, plus extra for dusting

· 2 teaspoons salt

· 2 teaspoons fast-action yeast

· 1½ cups cool water

Directions:

1.Oil a 2¼ liter square plastic container with olive oil.

2.Prepare a freestanding mixer with a dough hook and add salt, flour, and yeast to its bowl. Pour in the water (three-quarters) and start mixing at a slow speed. Gradually pour in the rest of the water when the dough comes together and mix for 5-7 minutes at a medium speed. You should get an elastic and glossy dough.

3.Transfer the dough to the oiled container, cover, and leave for 1 hour.

4.Dust a linen baker couche and the work surface with flour. Gently place your dough onto the work surface.

5.Divide it evenly into 4 portions. Flatten the dough and fold its sides to the center to form an oblong from each piece. Roll every piece up into a sausage with a smooth top and join through the whole length of the base. Starting from the middle, roll each piece with both hands. Make a forward and backward movement without heavy pressing to roll out 1½" long baguettes.

6.Place a baguette along the edge of the couche and pleat it up against the edge of the bread. Repeat for all of the baguettes—they should be lined up against each other and divided with a pleat between each. Cover with a tea towel and leave for 1 hour to double in size.

7.Preheat the oven to 465° F and put a roasting tray in the bottom.

8.When the dough has doubled in size, put them on the work surface, and dust it with flour. Make four slashes along the length of the baguette with a sharp knife. Place each baguette on a baking tray.

9.Put the bread into the oven and pour the hot water on the roasting tray for steam. Close the oven and bake for 10-20 minutes or longer for a deep color.

10. Take out of the oven and let the baguettes cool completely before slicing.

Nutrition:

· Calories: 170

· Carbohydrates:18 g

· Fat:0 g

Whole-Wheat Baguette

Preparation Time: 2 h 40 min.

2 -Pound Loaf

Ingredients:

· 3 cups warm water 80°F

· 1½ tablespoons granulated yeast

· 1½ tablespoons kosher salt

· 2½ cups ground hard white wheat flour

· 4 cups all-purpose flour

Directions:

1.Mix the yeast, water, and salt in a large bowl. Combine the flours in another bowl and mix well. Add the mixed flour to a bowl with water and stir with a wooden spoon. Knead with your hands if it's hard to stir. Cover with plastic wrap and leave for 4-5 hours until it begins to flatten on top.

2.Preheat the oven to 450° F. Place a baking stone on the central oven rack and a cast-iron skillet on a lower shelf.

3.Dust the dough top with flour and cut off a 1lb portion. Return the rested dough to the fridge.

4.Dust your dough lightly with flour and form into a ball. When it's cohesive, stretch and elongate it to create a cylinder (2" in diameter). Dust a piece of the parchment with whole wheat flour. Transfer the pound onto the paper and leave for 1 minute.

5.Next, lightly dampen the surface of the pound. Make a few diagonal slashes across the top of the baguette with a serrated bread knife.

6. Transfer it onto the hot stone and pour 1 cup of hot water into the skillet. Close the oven and bake for 25 minutes or longer to get the deep brown crust.

7.Remove and let it cool for 40 minutes before slicing.

Nutrition:

· Carbohydrates: 5 g Fat: 00 g Protein: 2 g

· Calories: 169 Sodium: 360 mg

Gluten-Free French Baguette

Preparation Time: 10 min. + 1 h.

1- Pound Loaf

Ingredients:

· 1 cup gluten-free white rice flour

· ½ cup arrowroot flour

· 1½ teaspoons Xanthan gum

· ¾ teaspoon Himalayan fine salt

· ¾ cup warm water

· 1 tablespoon pure maple syrup

· 2 ¼ teaspoons gluten-free active dry yeast

· 1 tablespoon extra virgin olive oil + some for brushing

· 2 large egg whites, at room temperature, whisked

· ½ teaspoon apple cider vinegar

Directions:

1.Mix all of the dry ingredients in a large bowl.

2.Mix the water, maple syrup, and yeast in another bowl. Leave it for 5minutes until the yeast foams.

3.Add the olive oil, yeast, egg whites, and vinegar to the dry mixture. Beat for 1 minute with a mixer. Scrape the sides while mixing.

4.Put your dough onto a greased French bread pan and spoon with olive oil. Make a few slashes diagonally and brush with olive oil. Cover tightly with a kitchen towel and leave for 40 minutes in a warm place.

5.Preheat the oven to 400°F and transfer the dough into it. Bake for 35-40 minutes until it has a nice golden crust.

6.Take out from the oven and let it cool for 40 minutes before slicing.

Nutrition:

· Calories: 181

· Carbohydrates: 15 g

· Fat: 2 g

· Protein: 2 g

· Sodium: 170 mg

Seeded Pumpkin Baguette

Preparation Time: 10 min. + 1h. 30 min.

1-Pound Loaf

Ingredients:

For the bread:

· 1½ cups pumpkin puree

· 2 teaspoons instant yeast

· 2 teaspoons honey

· ½ cup lukewarm water

· 2 teaspoons vegetable oil

· 3½ cups all-purpose flour

· ½ cup sunflower seeds

· 2 teaspoons sesame seeds

· 1 tablespoon flax seeds

· 2 teaspoons salt

For the topping:

· 1 egg lightly beaten

· ¼ cup pepitas pumpkin seeds

· 1 tablespoon poppy seeds

· 2 tablespoons sunflower seeds

Directions:

1. In the stand mixer bowl (with paddle attachment) add the pumpkin puree, honey, yeast, water, oil, and 1 cup of flour. Mix well to combine at a low speed. Add the seeds and salt. Then, set the kneading hook. Slowly add in 2 cups of flour, kneading until fully incorporated. Add more flour if you still haven't got a moist and smooth dough. Transfer the dough to a well-oiled bowl, cover with plastic wrap and leave for 60-90 minutes to rise.

2. Place dough onto a floured surface and carefully deflate. Then, divide the dough evenly into 6 pieces and form each one into a 1½" wide and 1½" long log. Transfer them onto a large greased baking sheet. Cover using a kitchen towel and leave for 30-45 minutes.

3. Preheat the oven to 400° F.

4. Brush your bread with beaten egg and sprinkle with sunflower seeds, pepitas, and poppy seeds.

5. Bake for 25 minutes or longer to get a deeper crust.

6. Take the baguettes out of the oven and allow them to completely cool on a cooling rack.

Nutrition:

· Calories: 229

· Carbohydrates:15g

· Fat:17 g

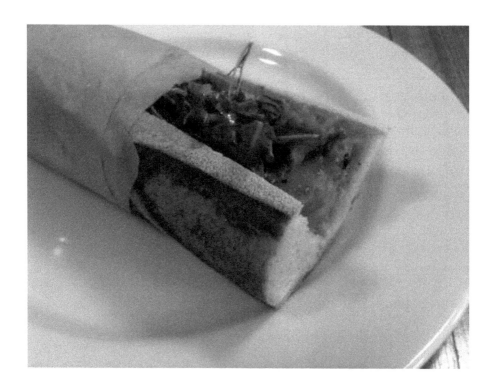

Wheat Shaft Baguette

Preparation Time: 1 min. + 2 h.

3-Pound Loaf

Ingredients:

· 1½ tablespoons granulated yeast

· 1½ tablespoons kosher salt

· 3 cups lukewarm water

· 6½ cups bread flour, plus more for the work surface and shaping

Directions:

1. Mix the yeast, water, and salt in a large bowl. Add the flour and mix with a stand mixer (paddle attachment). Cover using a kitchen towel and leave for 2 hours to double in size.

2. Next, flour the surface of the dough and cut off a ½-pound portion. Flour a piece of dough and form a ball: stretch its surface around the bottom while rotating the dough a quarter-turn as you go. Leave the dough for 5 minutes.

3. Form a rectangle of sorts from the ball. Next, using the palms of your hands, carefully roll it into a 1¼" baguette. Save the rest of the unused dough in the fridge. Turn over the baking sheet and line it with parchment paper. Transfer your dough onto it and leave for 40 minutes to rise.

4.Put another baking sheet in the middle of the oven and roasting pan in the bottom of the oven. Preheat it to 450° F.

5.Dust your dough with flour. Cover the blades of your kitchen scissors with oil and cut into the dough crosswise near the top of the baguette shape, at an angle of 25° to the dough and stopping a quarter inch from its bottom. Fold every cut part over to the side while alternating sides with every cut. Repeat to cut the entire pound.

6.Gently transfer the pound onto the baking sheet and pour 1 cup of hot water into the pan. Close the oven and bake for 25-30 minutes or longer for a deeper color.

7.Remove the baguette from the oven and let it cool completely before serving.

Nutrition:

· Calories: 234

· Carbohydrates: 46 g

· Fat: 1 g

· Protein: 1½ g

· Sodium: 350 mg

Classic Ciabatta

Preparation Time: 10 minutes + 1½ hours

2-Pound Loaf

Ingredients:

· 3½ cups unbleached, unbromated white bread flour

· 1½ teaspoons fine sea salt

· 1 teaspoon instant dry yeast

· 1½ cups warm water 65°F, + 2 teaspoons water

· 1 tablespoon extra-virgin olive oil

Directions:

1.Mix the yeast, flour, and salt in a large bowl, add half of the water into the mixer bowl (using the dough hook). Add all of the dry ingredients and mix at a low speed. Quickly pour in enough of the rest of the water in a slow stream to get a soft and moist dough. Stop mixing and scrape down the hook and the sides of the bowl with a spatula. Mix for 5 more minutes when you've added all the water.

2.Next, mix for 4 minutes on a medium-low speed while adding 1 tsp of olive oil. Mix for 1 more minute until the oil has been fully incorporated. The dough should be smooth and soft with a moist surface. Cover and leave for 3 hours, with a fold after each hour.

3.Oil a large bowl with extra olive oil and put your dough into it. Using your hands, pull one edge, fold it to the center, and lightly press down. Turn the bowl and repeat for the rest of the edges to form a ball. Turn the ball in the bowl to coat it with oil. Leave the dough for 3 hours, folding each hour.

4.Flour a work surface well. Dust the top of the dough and place it onto the work surface. Lightly dust all the sides of the dough and let it rest for 30 seconds.

5.Form a large rectangle from the dough. Put it in a floured couche and cover. Leave for 45-60 minutes, but keep an eye on the dough and determine whether it is ready to be baked. With your fingertip, make dents in the center of the dough. If it slowly and evenly disappears, you can bake it.

6.Put a baking stone on the bottom rack and preheat the oven to 450° F.

7.Line a bread peel with parchment paper. Transfer the bread to the peel, top side up. Place the dough on the parchment paper onto the middle of the stone. Cover it with a large stainless-steel bowl and close the oven. Bake for 5minutes then remove the bowl. Bake for 15 more minutes to get a golden ciabatta.

8.Take out of the oven and put the ciabatta on a cooling rack. Let it cool completely before slicing.

Nutrition:

· Calories: 169

· Carbohydrates: 25 g

· Fat:1 g

No-Knead Ciabatta

Preparation Time: 10 minutes + 11 ½ h.

2 -Pound Loaf

Ingredients:

· 4 cups unbleached all-purpose flour

· 1½ teaspoons kosher salt

· ¼ teaspoon active dry yeast

· 2 cups water

· 1 tablespoon olive oil

· 2 tablespoons cornmeal

Directions:

1.Mix the yeast, flour, and salt in a large bowl. Add the water and mix well, using a rubber spatula. Cover with foil and leave for 11 ½ hours at room temperature.

2.Next, oil a rimmed baking sheet with a brush, dust with cornmeal and set aside.

3.Wipe the work surface with water and line it with a piece of plastic wrap. Flour it to prevent the dough from sticking.

4.Place your dough onto the floured plastic wrap. Press and form a long flat pound from the dough. Next, flip your dough over on the prepared sheet pan using the plastic wrap. Lightly dust the top of the ciabatta with flour and cover with a kitchen towel for 2 hours.

5.Preheat the oven to 425° F. Put the rack in the lower third position. When it's preheated, transfer the sheet pan into the oven. Bake for 25-30 minutes or more until you get a beautiful deep golden crust.

6.Remove from the oven and let the ciabatta to cool completely before slicing on a cooling

7.rack.

Nutrition:

· Calories: 171

· Carbohydrates:8 g

· Fat:1 g

· Protein:2 g

· Sodium: 360 mg

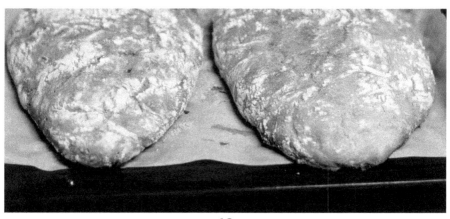

Quick Ciabatta

Preparation Time: 30 minutes + 3 hours.

2-Pound Loaf

Ingredients:

· 4 cups all-purpose flour

· 2¼ teaspoons active dry yeast

· 2¼ cups warm water

· 1 teaspoon salt

· ¼ teaspoon sugar

Directions:

1.Mix the yeast, sugar, and water in a mixing bowl and set aside for 5 minutes. Add the flour and salt and mix in a stand mixer with a paddle. You should get almost a pancake batter, only thicker.

2.Let it stand for 15 minutes. Then mix it at a medium-high speed for 6 minutes. Next, switch the paddle to the dough hook and mix for 6 more minutes to make the dough smooth and not sticking to the bowl.

3.Grease another bowl with oil and put the dough inside. Cover using a kitchen towel and leave for 2 hours in a warm place to triple in size. While it's rising, line a baking sheet with parchment paper and then dust it with flour.

4.Place your dough on the center of the baking sheet and flour the top. Divide the dough evenly into two pieces with a bench scraper. Also, use it and wet hand to shape the dough-tuck every irregular part underneath to get two flat logs. The logs should be about 6" apart. Remember that wet dough doesn't hold a definite shape, so you don't need to shape it perfectly.

5.Dust the tops with flour and cover using a kitchen towel for 1 hour to rise.

6.Preheat your oven to 500°F, keeping the baking stone inside for 30 minutes. Place a pan on the bottom rack.

7.Place the loaves on the baking stone by sliding the parchment off the sheet and pour hot water into the pan, close the oven. Bake for 25 minutes or until the bread has a golden-brown color.

8.Remove from the oven and cool for 40 minutes before slicing.

Nutrition:

· Calories: 172

· Carbohydrates: 28 g

· Fat: 1 g

· Protein: 2 g

· Sodium: 240 mg

Whole-Wheat Ciabatta

Preparation Time: 45 minutes + overnight

1-Pound Loaf

Ingredients:

For the sponge:

· 1 cup warm water

· ½ cup all-purpose flour

· ½ cup whole wheat flour

· ¼ cup rye flour

· ¼ teaspoon active dry yeast

For the final dough:

· 1 cup all-purpose flour

· 1 cup whole wheat flour

· ½ cup water at room temperature

· 2 tablespoons shelled sunflower seeds

· 1 tablespoon polenta

· 1 tablespoon ground flax seeds

· 1¾ teaspoons salt - 1½ teaspoons honey

· 1 teaspoon all-purpose flour, or as needed

· ½ teaspoon cornmeal, or as needed

Directions:

1. Mix all of the sponge ingredients in a large mixing bowl. Cover with plastic wrap and leave for 5-6 hours to double in size.

2.Then, stir in all the ingredients for the final dough into the bowl with a sponge. Mix for 3-4 minutes with a wooden spoon until you get a sticky dough ball. Scrape down all sides of the bowl, cover again with plastic wrap, and leave overnight.

3.Line your baking sheet with parchment and dust it with ½ teaspoon all-purpose flour and cornmeal.

4.Transfer your dough onto the floured surface and press to deflate the air. Shape into a smooth rectangle pound. Transfer it onto the prepared baking sheet, lightly dust them and cover with plastic wrap for 1 hour and 30 minutes.

5.Preheat the oven to 450° F. Put a skillet on the bottom rack and pour 1 cup of hot water into it.

6.Lightly mist the top of the pound and put it into the oven. Bake for 30-35 minutes, dampening the top of the bread every 2 minutes. Remove your bread from the oven and cool completely on a cooling rack before slicing.

Nutrition:

· Calories: 185

· Carbohydrates: 26 g

Anadama Bread

Preparation Time: 1 hour

1½-PoundLoaf

Ingredients:

· 1 package (1/4oz.) active dry yeast

· 1 tablespoon sugar

· 1 cup warm water at 80°F

· 2 large eggs

· 3 tablespoons canola oil

· 1 tablespoon molasses

· 1 teaspoon white vinegar

· 1½ cups gluten-free all-purpose baking flour

· ¾ cup cornmeal

· 1½ teaspoons Xanthan gum

· ½ teaspoon salt

Direction:

1.Grease 1 ½ x 4-inch Pound pan. Sprinkle using gluten-free flour, put aside.

2.Melt sugar and yeast in warm water. Mix the vinegar, molasses, oil, and eggs in a stand mixer's bowl with a paddle attachment. Then add Whisk, Xanthan gum, cornmeal, and flour.

3.Beat for one minute on low speed, beat for two minutes on medium speed. The dough will be softer compared to yeast bread dough that has gluten. Put in a prepped pan, use a wet spatula to smooth the top. Rise with cover for 40 minutes until the dough reaches the pan's lid in a warm place.

4.Bake for 1 minute at 375° F, then loosely cover using foil. Bake till golden brown for 1¼ -15 minutes more, turn the oven off. In an oven, leave bread for 15 minutes with the door ajar. Transfer from pan onto a wire rack. Allow cooling.

Nutrition:

· Calories: 176

· Carbohydrates: 21 g

· Cholesterol: 35 mg

· Total Fat: 5 g

· Fiber: 3 g

· Protein: 4 g

· Sodium: 120 m

Sandwich Bread

Preparation Time: 1 hour

1-Pound Loaf

Ingredients:

· 1 tablespoon active dry yeast

· 2 tablespoons sugar

· 1 cup warm fat-free milk

· 2 egg whites

· 3 tablespoons canola oil

· 1 teaspoon cider vinegar

· 2½ cups gluten-free all-purpose baking flour

· 2½ teaspoons Xanthan gum

· 1 teaspoon unflavored gelatin

· ½ teaspoon salt

Direction:

1.Oil a pound pan, 9x5 inches in size, and dust with gluten-free flour reserve.

2.In warm milk, melt sugar and yeast in a small bowl—mix yeast mixture, vinegar, oil, and eggs in a stand with a paddle. Slowly whip in salt, gelatin, Xanthan gum, and flour. Whip for a minute on low speed. Whip for 2 minutes on moderate. The dough will become softer compared to the yeast bread dough that has gluten. Turn onto the prepped pan. Using a wet spatula, smoothen the surface. Put a cover and rise in a warm area for 25 minutes until dough extends to the pan top.

3.Bake for 1 minute at 375° F, loosely cover with foil. Bake till golden brown for 5 to 15 minutes more. Take out from pan onto a wire rack to let cool.

Nutrition:

· Calories: 195

· Carbohydrates: 17 g

· Cholesterol: 27 mg

· Total Fat: 4 g

· Fiber: 2 g

· Protein: 4 g

· Sodium: 120 mg

Rosemary Bread

Preparation Time: 10 minutes

1½- Pound Loaf

Ingredients:

· 1 ¼ cups warm water

· ¼ cup olive oil

· 2 egg whites

· 1 tablespoon apple cider vinegar

· ½ teaspoon baking powder

· 2 teaspoons dry active yeast

· 2 tablespoons granulated sugar

· ½ teaspoon Italian seasoning

· ¼ teaspoon ground black pepper

· 1¼ teaspoons dried rosemary

· 2 cups gluten-free almond flour / or any other gluten-free flour, leveled

· 1 cup tapioca/potato starch, leveled

· 2 teaspoons Xanthan Gum

· 1 teaspoon salt

Directions:

1.According to your bread machine manufacturer, place all the ingredients into the bread machine's greased pan.

2.Select basic cycle/standard cycle/bake/quick bread/white bread setting, then choose crust colour either medium or Light and press start to bake bread.

3.In the last kneading cycle, check the dough, it should be wet but thick, not like traditional bread dough. If the dough is too wet, put more flour, one tablespoon at a time, or until dough slightly firm.

4.When the cycle is finished, and the baker machine turns off, remove baked bread from pan and cool on wire rack.

Nutrition:

· Calories: 180

· Total fat: 3 g

· Protein:6g

· Cholesterol: 5 mg

· Sodium: 240 mg

· Carbohydrates: 24 g

· Fiber: 1 g

Flax and Sunflower Seeds Bread

Preparation Time: 10 minutes

2-Pound Loaf

Ingredients:

· 1¼ cups warm water

· ¼ cup olive oil

· 2 egg whites

· 1 tablespoon apple cider vinegar

· ½ teaspoon baking powder

· 2 teaspoons dry active yeast

· 2 tablespoons granulated sugar

· 2 cups gluten-free almond flour / or any other gluten-free flour, leveled

· 1 cup tapioca/potato starch, leveled

· 2 teaspoons Xanthan Gum

· 1 teaspoon salt

· ½ cup flax seeds

· ½ cup sunflower seeds

Directions:

1.According to your bread machine manufacturer, place all the ingredients into the bread machine's greased pan except sunflower seeds.

2.Select basic cycle/standard cycle/bake/quick bread/white bread setting, then select crust colour either medium or light and press start.

3.In the last kneading cycle, check the dough, it should be wet but thick, not like traditional bread dough. If the dough is too wet, put more flour, one tablespoon at a time, or until the dough slightly firm.

4.Add sunflower seeds 5 minutes before the kneading cycle ends.

5.When the cycle is finished and the machine turns off, remove baked bread from pan and cool on wire rack.

Nutrition:

· Calories: 190

· Total fat: 2g

· Cholesterol: 5 mg

· Sodium: 240 mg

· Carbohydrates: 21 g

· Fiber: 2 g

· Protein: 4 g

Italian Parmesan Cheese Bread

Preparation Time: 10 minutes

2-Pound Loaf

Inredients:

· 1¼ cups warm water

· ¼ cup olive oil

· 2 egg whites

· 1 tablespoon apple cider vinegar

· ½ teaspoon baking powder

· 2 teaspoons dry active yeast

· 2 tablespoons granulated sugar

· 2 cups gluten-free almond flour / or any other gluten-free flour, leveled

· 1 cup tapioca/potato starch, leveled

· 2 teaspoons Xanthan Gum

· ¼ cup grated Parmesan cheese

· 1 teaspoon salt

· 1 teaspoon Italian seasoning

· 1 teaspoon garlic powder

Directions:

1.According to your bread machine manufacturer, place all the ingredients into the bread machine's greased pan, and select a basic cycle/standard cycle/bake/quick bread/white bread setting. Then choose crust colour, either medium or light, and press start to bake bread.

2.In the last kneading cycle, check the dough, it should be wet but thick, not like traditional bread dough. If the dough is too wet, put more flour, one tablespoon at a time, or until the dough slightly firm.

3.When the cycle is finished and the machine turns off, remove baked bread from pan and cool on wire rack.

Nutrition:

· Calories: 190

· Total fat: 2 g

· Cholesterol: 2 mg

· Sodium: 240 mg

· Carbohydrates: 15 g

· Fiber: 1 g

· Protein: 2 g

Cheese & Herb Bread

Preparation Time: 10 minutes

2-Pound Loaf

Ingredients:

· 1¼ cups warm water

· ¼ cup olive oil

· 2 egg whites

· 1 tablespoon apple cider vinegar

· ½ teaspoon baking powder

· 2 teaspoons dry active yeast

· 2 tablespoons granulated sugar

· 2 cups gluten-free almond flour / or any other gluten-free flour, leveled

· 1 cup Tapioca/potato starch, leveled

· 2 teaspoons Xanthan Gum

· 1 teaspoon salt

· 2 tablespoons grated Parmesan cheese

· 1 teaspoon dried marjoram

· ¾ teaspoon dried basil

Directions:

1.According to your bread machine manufacturer, place all the ingredients into the bread machine's greased pan, and select a basic cycle/standard cycle/bake/quick bread/white bread setting. Then choose crust colour, either medium or light, and press start to bake bread.

2.In the last kneading cycle, check the dough, it should be wet but thick, not like traditional bread dough. If the dough is too wet, put more flour, one tablespoon at a time, or until the dough slightly firm.

3.When the cycle is finished and the machine turns off, remove baked bread from pan and cool on wire rack.

Nutrition:

· Calories: 230

· Total fat: 3 g

· Cholesterol: 5 mg

· Sodium: 245 mg

· Carbohydrates: 19 g

· Fiber: 1 g

· Protein: 4 g

Cinnamon Raisin Bread

Preparation Time: 15 minutes

2-Pound Loaf

Ingredients:

· 1¼ cups warm water

· ¼ cup olive oil

· 2 tablespoons honey

· 2 egg whites

· 1 tablespoon apple cider vinegar

· ½ teaspoon baking powder

· 2 teaspoons dry active yeast

· 2 tablespoons granulated sugar

· 2 cups gluten-free almond flour / or any other gluten-free flour, leveled

· 1 cup Tapioca/potato starch, leveled

· 2 teaspoons Xanthan Gum

· 1 teaspoon salt

· 1 teaspoon ground cinnamon

· 1 cup raisins

Directions:

1.According to your bread machine manufacturer, place all the ingredients into the bread machine's greased pan except raisins.

2.Select basic cycle/standard cycle/bake/quick bread/sweet bread setting, then choose crust colour either medium or Light and press start to bake bread.

3.In the last kneading cycle, check the dough, it should be wet but thick, not like traditional bread dough. If the dough is too wet, put more flour, one tablespoon at a time, or until dough slightly firm.

4.Add raisins 5 minutes before the kneading cycle ends.

5.When the cycle is finished and the machine turns off, remove baked bread from pan and cool on wire rack.

Nutrition:

· Calories: 219

· Fat: 1 g

· Cholesterol: 2 mg

· Sodium: 240 mg

· Carbohydrates: 22 g

Bakers Bread

Preparation Time: 1 hour

1-Pound Loaf

Ingredients:

· Pinch of salt

· 4 tablespoons light cream cheese softened

· ½ teaspoon cream of tartar

· 4 eggs, yolks, and whites separated

Directions:

1.Heat 2 racks in the middle of the oven at 350º F.

2.Line 2 baking pan with parchment paper, then grease with cooking spray.

3.Separate egg yolks from the whites and place them in separate mixing bowls.

4.Beat the egg whites and cream of tartar with a hand mixer until stiff, about 3 to 5 minutes. Do not over-beat.

5.Whisk the cream cheese, salt, and egg yolks until smooth.

6.Slowly fold the cheese mix into the whites until fluffy.

7.Spoon ¼ cup measure of the batter onto the baking sheets, 6 mounds on each sheet.

8.Bake in the oven for 1 to 22 minutes, alternating racks halfway through.

9. Cool and serve.

Nutrition:

· Calories: 191

· Fat: 3.2 g

· Carbohydrates:1 g

· Protein: 2.4 g

· Sodium: 30 mg

Bulgur Bread

Preparation Time: 15 minutes

1½-Pound Loaf

Ingredients:

· ½ cup bulgur

· 1/3 cup boiling water

· 1 egg

· 1 cup water

· 1 tablespoon butter

· 1½ tablespoons milk powder

· 1 tablespoon sugar

· 2 teaspoons salt

· 3¼ cup flour

· 1 teaspoon dried yeast

Directions:

1.Bulgur pour boiling water into a small container and cover with a lid. Leave to stand for 30 minutes.

2.Cut butter into small cubes.

3.Stir the egg with water in a measuring container. The total volume of eggs with water should be 300 ml.

4.Put all the ingredients in the bread maker in the order that is described in the instructions for your bread maker. Bake in the basic mode, medium crust.

Nutrition:

· Calories: 255

· Carbohydrates: 3 g

· Fats: 3 g

· Protein: 1½ g

· Sodium: 480 mg

· Fiber: 1.2 g

Almond Meal Bread

Preparation Time: 1 hour

1-Pound Loaf

Ingredients:

· 4 eggs, pasteurized

· ¼ cup melted coconut oil

· 1 tablespoon apple cider vinegar

· 2¼ cups almond meal

· 1 teaspoon baking soda

· ¼ cup ground flaxseed meal

· 1 teaspoon onion powder

· 1 tablespoon minced garlic

· 1 teaspoon of sea salt

· 1 teaspoon chopped sage leaves

· 1 teaspoon fresh thyme

· 1 teaspoon chopped rosemary leaves

Directions:

1.Gather all the ingredients for the bread and plug in the bread machine having the capacity of 2 pounds of bread recipe.

2.Take a large bowl, crack eggs in it and then beat in coconut oil and vinegar until well blended.

3. Take a separate large bowl, place the almond meal in it, add remaining ingredients, and stir until well mixed.

4.Add egg mixture into the bread bucket, top with flour mixture, shut the lid, select the "basic/white" cycle or "low-carb" setting and then press the up/down arrow button to adjust baking time according to your bread machine; it will take 3 to 4 hours.

5.Then press the crust button to select light crust if available, and press the "start/stop" button to switch on the bread machine.

6.When the bread machine beeps, open the lid, then take out the bread basket and lift out the bread.

7.Let bread cool on a wire rack for 1 hour, then cut it into ten pounds and serve.

Nutrition:

· Calories: 194

· Sodium: 240 mg

· Fat: 2 g

· Protein: 4 g

· Carbohydrates: 2.1 g

· Fiber: 2 g

· Net Carbohydrates: 0.3 g

Italian Blue Cheese Bread

Preparation Time: 3 hours

1½-Pound Loaf

Ingredients:

· 1 teaspoon dry yeast

· 2½ cups almond flour

· 1½ teaspoon salt

· 1 tablespoon sugar

· 1 tablespoon olive oil

· ½ cup blue cheese

· 1 cup water

Directions:

1.Mix all the ingredients.

2.Start baking.

3.When the cycle is finished and the machine turns off, remove baked bread from pan and cool on wire rack.

Nutrition:

· Calories: 194

· Carbohydrates 5 g

· Fats 4.6 g

· Protein: 6 g

· Fiber: 1.5 g

· Sodium: 360 mg

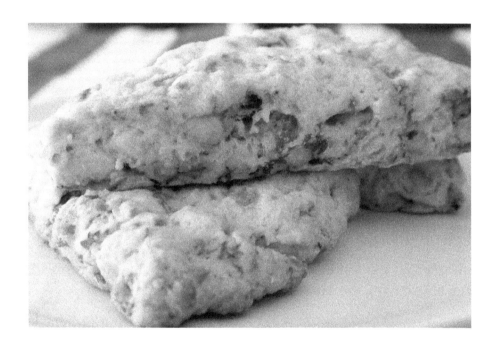

Macadamia Nut Bread

Preparation Time: 10 minutes

1½-Pound Loaf

Ingredients:

· 1 cup / 135 grams macadamia nuts

· 5 eggs, pasteurized

· 1 cup water

· ½ teaspoon apple cider vinegar

· ¼ cup / 30 grams coconut flour

· ½ teaspoon baking soda

Directions:

1.Gather all the ingredients for the bread and plug in the bread machine having the capacity of 1 pound of bread recipe.

2.Place nuts in a blender, pulse for 2 to 3 minutes until mixture reaches a consistency of butter, and then blend in eggs and vinegar until smooth.

3.Stir in flour and baking soda until well mixed.

4.Add the batter into the bread bucket, shut the lid, select the "basic/white" cycle or "low-carb" setting and then press the up/down arrow button to adjust baking time according to your bread machine; it will take 3 to 4 hours.

5.Then press the crust button to select light crust if available, and press the "start/stop" button to switch on the bread machine.

6.When the bread machine beeps, open the lid, then take out the bread basket and lift out the bread.

7.Let bread cool on a wire rack for 1 hour, then cut it into eight pounds and serve.

Nutrition:

· Calories: 175

· Sodium: 20 mg

· Fat: 1.3 g

· Protein: 5.6 g

· Carbohydrates: 3.9 g

· Fiber: 3 g

· Net Carbohydrates: 0.9 g

Cheesy Garlic Bread

Preparation Time: 1 hour

2-Pound Loaf

Ingredients:

For the Bread:

· 5 eggs, pasteurized

· 1 cup water

· 2 cups / 10 grams almond flour

· ½ teaspoon Xanthan gum

· 1 teaspoon garlic powder

· 1 teaspoon salt

· 1 teaspoon parsley

· 1 teaspoon Italian seasoning

· 1 teaspoon dried oregano

· 1 stick of butter, grass-fed, unsalted, melted

· 1 cup grated mozzarella cheese

· 2 tablespoons ricotta cheese

· 1 cup / 235 grams grated cheddar cheese

· 1/3 cup / 30 grams grated parmesan cheese

For the Topping:

· ½ stick of butter, grass-fed, unsalted, melted

· 1 teaspoon garlic powder

Directions:

1.Gather all the ingredients for the bread and plug in the bread machine having the capacity of 2 pounds of bread recipe.

2.Take a large bowl, crack eggs in it and then whisk until blended.

3.Take a separate large bowl, place flour in it, and stir in Xanthan gum and all the cheeses until well combined.

4.Take a medium bowl, place butter in it, add all the seasonings in it, and stir until mixed.

5.Add egg mixture into the bread bucket, top with seasoning mixture and flour mixture, shut the lid, select the "basic/white" cycle or "low-carb" setting and then press the up/down arrow button to adjust baking time according to your bread machine; it will take 3 to 4 hours.

6.Then press the crust button to select light crust if available, and press the "start/stop" button to switch on the bread machine.

7.When the bread machine beeps, open the lid, then take out the bread basket and lift out the bread.

8.Prepare the topping by mixing together melted butter and garlic powder and brush the mixture on top of the bread.

9.Let bread cool on a wire rack for 1 hour, then cut it into sixteen pounds and serve.

Nutrition:

· Calories: 250

· Fat: 1.5 g

· Sodium: 400 mg

· Protein: 7.2 g

· Carbohydrates: 3 g

· Fiber: 1.6 g

· Net Carbohydrates: 1.4 g

Almond Pumpkin Quick Bread

Preparation Time: 35 minutes

1½-Pound Loaf

Ingredients

· 1/3 cup vegetable oil

· ½ cup water

· 3 large eggs

· 1 ½ cups pumpkin puree, canned

· 1 cup granulated sugar

· 1½ teaspoons baking powder

· ½ teaspoon baking soda

· ¼ teaspoon salt

· ¾ teaspoon ground cinnamon

· ¼ teaspoon ground nutmeg

· ¼ teaspoon ground ginger

· 3 cups almond flour

· ½ cup chopped pecans

Directions

1.Spray your bread machine pan with cooking spray.

2.In a bowl, mix all the wet ingredients until blended. Add all the dry ingredients except pecans until mixed.

3.Pour the batter onto your bread machine pan and place it back inside the bread machine. Close the cover securely.

4.Turn on the bread machine and select QUICK BREAD cycle then press START.

5.When your bread machine pings, pause and open the lid then add the chopped pecans. Then close the lid and press START to let the cycle continue.

6.Once cycle is finished, loosen the pound from the pan and transfer to a cooling rack.

7.Slice and serve with your favorite keto soup.

Nutrition:

· Calories: 250

· Sodium: 70 mg

· Fat: 1.5 g

· Protein: 7.2 g

· Carbohydrates: 3 g

· Fiber: 1.6 g

· Net Carbohydrates: 1.4 g

Basil Parmesan Slices

Preparation Time: 10 minutes

Cooking Time: 2 hour s

1½-Pound loaf

Ingredients:

· 1 cup water

· ½ cup parmesan cheese, grated

· 3 tablespoons sugar

· 1 tablespoon dried basil

· 1½ tablespoons olive oil

· 1 teaspoon salt

· 3 cups almond flour

· 2 teaspoons active dry yeast

Directions:

1.Place all the ingredients in your bread machine pan according to the list stated in the ingredients list.

2.Close the lid then set the bread machine on BASIC cycle and press START.

3.Once the cycle is done, move pound to a cooling rack.

4.Slice and serve as a side dish for your soup or main course.

Nutrition:

· Calories: 250

· Sodium: 240 mg

· Fat: 1.5 g

· Protein: 7.2 g

· Carbohydrates: 3 g

· Fiber: 1.6 g

· Net Carbohydrates: 1.4 g

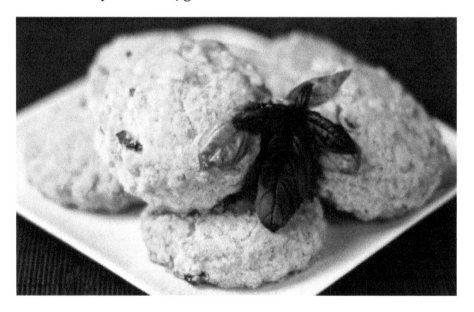

Onion Bread

Preparation Time: 45 minutes

2-Pound Loaf

Ingredients:

· 1½ cups water

· 2 tablespoons + 2 teaspoons butter, unsalted

· 1½ teaspoons salt

· 1 tablespoon + 1 teaspoon sugar

· 2 tablespoons + 2 teaspoons non-fat dry milk

· 4 cups almond flour

· 2 teaspoons active dry yeast

· 4 tablespoons dry onion soup mix

Directions:

1.Add all ingredients except dry onion mix in the bread machine pan according to the list above.

2.Close the lid cover. Select BASIC cycle on your bread machine and then press START.

3.Your machine will ping after around 30 to 40 minutes. This is your signal to add whatever fruit, nut, or flavoring you wish to add to your dough. Pause your bread machine and add the dry onion soup mix.

4.Press START again and allow the cycle to continue.

5.Once your pound is finished, transfer it to a cooling rack.

6. Slice and serve with cream cheese or butter or as a soup side dish.

Nutrition:

· Calories: 250

· Sodium: 360 mg

· Fat: 1.5 g Protein: 7.2 g

· Carbohydrates: 3 g

· Fiber: 1.6 g

Sundried Tomato Quick Bread

Preparation Time: 25 minutes

1½-Pound Loaf

Ingredients :

· 2¼ cups almond flour

· ½ water

· 1 tablespoon baking powder

· 1 teaspoon kosher salt

· 3 large eggs

· 1½ cups buttermilk

· 6 tablespoons canola oil

· 1 tablespoon dried basil

· 1 cup sundried tomato roughly chopped

Directions:

1.Place all the ingredients in your bread machine bucket except for basil and sundried tomato.

2.Secure the lid cover. Select the QUICK BREAD setting on your bread machine then press START.

3.Wait for the ping or the fruit and nut signal to open the lid and add the basil and sundried tomato. Close the lid again and press START to continue.

4.When the cycle finishes, transfer the pound to a wire rack and let it cool.

5. Slice and serve.

Nutrition:

· Calories: 250

· Sodium: 230 mg

· Fat: 1.5 g

· Protein: 7.2 g

· Carbohydrates: 3 g

· Fiber: 1.6 g

· Net Carbohydrates: 1.4 g

Cheddar Bacon and Chive Bread

Preparation Time: 10 minutes

1½-Pound Loaf

Ingredients

· 2¼ cups almond flour

· ½ water

· 1 tablespoon baking powder

· 1 teaspoon kosher salt

· 3 large eggs

· 1½ cups buttermilk

· 6 tablespoons canola oil

· 3 tablespoons finely chopped chives

· 1 cup shredded cheddar sharp cheese

· 6 strips bacon cook and crumbled

Directions:

1.Place all the ingredients in your bread machine bucket pan except for bacon.

2.Close the cover. Select the QUICK BREAD setting on your bread machine then press START.

3.Wait for the fruit and nut signal. Pause and open the lid and add the bacon. Close the lid again and press START to continue.

4.When the cycle finishes, transfer the pound to a wire rack and let it cool.

5.Slice and serve.

Nutrition:

· Calories: 250

· Sodium: 270 mg

· Fat: 1.5 g

· Protein: 7.2 g

· Carbohydrates: 3 g

· Fiber: 1.6 g

· Net Carbohydrates: 1.4 g

Tortilla Wraps

Preparation Time: 50 minutes

1-Pound Loaf

Ingredients

· 1 cup golden flaxseed meal

· 2 tablespoons coconut flour

· ½ teaspoon Xanthan gum

· ½ teaspoon salt

· 1 tablespoon butter

· 1 cup warm water

Directions

1.Add all ingredients into your bread machine. Close the lid cover.

2.Select DOUGH cycle and press START.

3.Once the cycle is finished, remove the dough and transfer it to a lightly floured working table.

4.Divide the dough into equal chunks. Roll out the dough into a thin shape.

5.On a skillet over low heat, cook the tortilla for 1-2 minutes each tortilla. Remove from the skillet and cover with a towel. The tortillas should be soft and not stiff.

6.Serve with your favorite filling.

Nutrition:

· Calories: 250

· Sodium: 130 mg

· Fat: 1.5 g

· Protein: 7.2 g

· Carbohydrates: 3 g

· Fiber: 1.6 g

· Net Carbohydrates: 1.4 g

Lightning Source UK Ltd.
Milton Keynes UK
UKHW020741250621
386134UK00001B/77